Masters of the Spirit World

HEALING

with the Universe, Meditation, and Prayer

Compiled by
Peter Watson Jenkins

Channeled by
Toni Ann Winninger

~Celestial Voices, Inc.~

Healing with The Universe, Meditation, and Prayer

Cover design by Robert Buzek Designs, Inc., Lake Zurich, Illinois

Published by Celestial Voices, Inc.,
7020 N. Wolcott Avenue, Chicago, Illinois 60626-2312.

ISBN: 978-0-9798917-0-0

FIRST EDITION

Printed in the United States of America

Important Note

The information contained in this book is intended
to be educational information only and not for the
diagnosis, prescription, or treatment of any medical
or psychological condition. If you need medical
advice you should contact a licensed healthcare
professional. The authors and publishers are in no
way liable for the misuse of this material..

Contents

Introducing the Masters   5
To Skeptics   9
Comment   13
Background Explanations:
   1. Incarnation   15
   2. Soul and Body   19
Section I
Healing with the Universe
   1. Getting Sick   23
   2. Getting Well   29
   3. Healing Therapies   34
   4. Weight Loss   45
The Soul's Creative Power   53
Comment   57
Section II
On Meditation   61
On Prayer   63
Prayer in the Christian Bible   73
Comment   90
The Authors   95

Acknowledgements

To Sonia A. Ness
for editing the manuscript.

To Robert Buzek
for designing the cover.

The Masters' Website

The Masters invite you to visit their website
to view their regular weekly messages:

www.MastersOfTheSpiritWorld.com

Introducing The Masters

Toni Ann Winninger and Peter Watson Jenkins have been working together with the Masters of the Spirit World since 2004.

Just as Toni, an attorney, was about to retire from her job as a prosecutor in the Chicago area, the Masters invited her to become a channeler. Toni was already well aware of her psychic abilities, knew that it was a big step for her to undertake, and did so quite tentatively at first.

Peter was one of the people who helped her develop her new-found channeling skill. He is an author and clinical hypnotist who had previously spent 21 years in parish ministry, mostly in Britain. Since then they have been working together with the Masters on hypnosis projects and channeled books.

The Masters are a large group of senior souls, many of whom have "ascended." This means that, having had many lives on Earth, they have completed their human lessons, gained enlightenment, and now, as mature spirits, are engaged in advising other souls. However, this is a large group and it also includes several angels, who we are told are souls who have never incarnated.

The Masters are thoughtful and wise with a tremendous sense of humor. Frequently wisecracks are traded with Peter and Toni just before the work begins on writing their books, a trilogy of interviews with 15 leaders of the past and with 42 twentieth-century celebrities.

Some time ago, Toni began referring to the group collectively as "The Guys." This does not mean to imply that all these souls are masculine, because all incarnating souls, who are inherently gender free, have spent some time living both in male and in female bodies. There's not the least bit of disrespect in our familiarity but simply recognition that all souls, including your own, are created equal by the Creator, in whose energy we all share. The Guys also seem to rather enjoy the modern, casual form of address.

The contents of this book demand that we try to understand how the Masters have a different way of looking at our life here on planet Earth. As Albert Einstein discovered, everything is composed of energy, so the Masters think of the world and of human beings in terms of our energy and of the vibrational level at which we function. They see the big picture of the universe in a way that we human beings cannot completely comprehend. Most importantly, they value everything in relation to the unconditional love and service of the spiritual Home where they live now, and to which we shall all return when our life here on planet Earth is over. Please take time to thoroughly digest the Masters' thoughts. The transcript of their words was carefully double checked with them to ensure that it is free from the bias of our opinion, and that it clearly and accurately presents the thoughts of the Masters themselves.

As we read the Masters' commentary, we need to understand that planet Earth is one place to which our souls migrate in order to learn by every single experience we have to face during physical life as human beings. The lessons are all pre-planned, experiences that have been chosen by each individual soul in order to further its personal growth and maturity.

Many of these lessons come though our varied experience of disease and pain, daily challenges for us to cope with, such as colds, obesity, anorexia, depression, cancer, and a host of physical traumas and accidents.

To face our experience of disease, many of us naturally resort to doctors and healers for practical help. Coping with such difficult challenges leads people to seek inner peace and to find spiritual answers to life's many problems, so we meditate and pray, both for ourselves and to help others in distress. The Masters give important new directions to our thinking about these issues and personal challenges.

Note

In the book, *Peter's questions and statements are printed in italic type.* The Masters' replies, and our concluding commentaries are all printed in roman type.

To Skeptics

What do you have to say to skeptics who read this channeled book?

We enjoy the stimulation that you provide for us because, without your questions, without your doubts, those involved in these messages would become complacent. It is your stimulation that makes us explain things that often appear to us as everyday occurrences, so we honor you in forcing us to do our work properly.

Our work is to let those in human form fully appreciate the possibilities of this type of communication and also to be able to communicate with us at will, so that we may assist them as they continue their journey through life. We have been their friends, acquaintances, and teachers in the past, and we simply wish to continue helping "from the wings" while they are in human form. To the skeptic we say that we are the guides, the directors, the prompters, who are here to be taken advantage of and used...but only if desired.

So you don't judge skeptics for being skeptics?
Absolutely not! The human experience is made for people to learn, to feel what it is like to be human, which is in a body that is solid and in a lot of cases impenetrable. You are like a machine that has endless amounts of data available for input. Based upon the data source, you have ocular inputs—eyes that gather various types of information. You have auditory inputs—ears that allow you to listen to what is being said as well. All this data must be processed internally. Most humans do this only with the brain, an unemotional machine. But your feeling heart is a center point within which you may remember whatever part you have played in the past in your non-physical life. So skepticism is just a natural initial stage within this data-gathering process.

This all seems rather like an argument for religion.
We beg to differ. Religion, as most people view it upon your planet, is a construct in which a person or group of people tell you what you must think, how you must behave—all in order to save your eternal soul. Then you must do what *they* think and what *they* say or you will be forever condemned to the eternal fires of hell.

So what's the point of reading your statements?
We present to each alive and thinking being upon the planet a kind of starter kit showing how to go inside and connect with (what even all the religions tell you exists) your soul. We define the soul as the energy within you which is the same as the energy that is in everyone else, because it all comes from a single source. That Source, the Creator, can be tapped in order to access the wisdom that has been gathered by all those who have lived before you, and by all the means you have used in your own previous learning experiences.

Now you really do sound religious, talking about a Creator. Can you prove the existence of God?

No. We're never going to be able to prove that to anyone while they are in physical form. That may seem to be the torpedo that sinks our boat. But on the other side of the coin, in response, we ask you to tell us about your origin, how you got here. Describe the power which is the force inside of you. Go back to the very first organism that resulted in your species. Granted, you can show us a lineage of biological people related to you in that physical form, but go beyond them—where did they come from? How did they get here? How did the planet beneath your feet come into existence? What? Did we hear you say someone must have created them? Our point exactly!

~.~

"We thank you because we quite enjoy the stimulation that you provide for us."

The Masters

Comment

Some people may greet the words from our friends on the other side with difficulty and genuine skepticism. Peter and Toni can provide no proof of the authenticity of the Masters themselves except for our strong inner conviction that they are loving spirits of the God-Force, and also because of the way in which, time after time, their words confirm what has been learned by spiritual people elsewhere.

Those who may ask whether this is an attempt to create a new dogma or a new religion should relax. Peter and Toni are absolutely clear that they are not promoting a new religious philosophy. They see themselves merely providing an outlet ("a voice") for the Masters, as requested. Every interpretation made here is given only to render more distinct the careful words which come from the higher dimension of the loving and caring Masters of the Spirit World.

We ask that you simply keep an open mind, not trying to analyze to death the concepts presented, but just allowing yourself see how the Masters' words *feel* to you.

To start off we have asked the Masters to provide some background information on the way in which souls come down to Earth in order to learn lessons through the varied experiences that living on our polarized planet affords. In their answer the Masters show how souls have access to a universal information database that our conscious mind knows little about initially, but which, in due course, as we become more fully aware of our soul and its purpose, we will increasingly become able to access.

Background Explanations

1. Incarnation

Masters, please explain the process of incarnation.

Broken off from the Creator, each soul is an energy capable of living in many different organisms. To experience something each soul must have the vehicle of a body *shell*. With its advisors, each soul decides what it wants to experience within the life-span of that body. It chooses its new parents. This will allow it to be placed in a suitable situation for whatever it has decided to experience in that life.

For example, should the soul want to experience grief, it will choose a family in which there is going to be a physical loss. So the soul may choose to inhabit the fetus that occurs from the union of those two parents. Generally, it is more convenient for it not to inhabit the growing organism until the fetus is near to birth, but it remains

15

close, monitoring what is going on. Sometimes, because the parents have freedom of choice, the baby's situation may change. There may be a stillbirth, or some anomaly, so that which is delivered does not need the soul, which will usually return Home.

When does the soul connect with the fetus?

Although a soul need not choose to enter a fetus fully until it is being born, it must make a light connection in order for the fetus to live. At the moment of conception there is a decision made by each soul that that unique fetus is in fact the chosen one. That is not a connection but an energetic acknowledgement. The soul is also aware of the act of conception. The soul may, in fact, be acting in cooperation with the biological parents to give the urge for the conception at a moment of its choosing. It is the soul who actually determines whether it wants the child to be male or female.

How does the soul actually inhabit the physical body?

It goes into the fetus, bringing with it the knowledge of its prior experiences. It enters everything, like a liquid totally saturating a piece of material. It is completely absorbed and becomes everything that is within the body of the fetus.

Then the memories of the soul are downloaded progressively. The soul is still free while the fetus, whose physical DNA is gradually being filled up, is becoming a storehouse of the knowledge and experience that the soul has had in its prior lives. Then all of the soul's memories and lessons (including the knowledge of whatever the soul needs to accomplish in the current incarnation), are contained within the host.

At what point does the total connection take place?

There is no set format. Less-mature souls might enter the fetus almost at the point of conception. More-experienced souls watch and wait outside before becoming a part of the baby when it is ready to be delivered. A small part of the soul is left at Home, in the spirit world, but the majority of the energy is put into the learning experience.

Can a child live without a soul?

For the baby to live apart from the mother, the soul must be inside. The idea that the baby is delivered and then the soul inhabits it is incorrect because the *shell* (body) would then die. It is very rare for the connection between soul and fetus ever to take place after the birth. Incorrect readings of this process may have come from the fact that it takes a while for the host to become used to the soul's energy, and to be aware of the point when the two became united.

Who makes the decision concerning the child's gender?

The decision concerning gender, which is made before the joining of egg and sperm, is the responsibility of the incarnating soul, not of the parents. The soul has complete freedom of choice when and how to come down to planet Earth. Gender, sexual orientation, and trans-sexuality are all types of lessons the soul wishes to experience.

The soul of a homosexual person, for instance, is not wanting to be the other sex, but rather needs experience of ambivalence, prejudice, and self-worth issues.

2. Soul and Body

Is incarnation about experiencing new feelings?

The soul connects with the body to experience physicality. Souls come down primarily to learn lessons, and then, while in the process of learning or after having learned those lessons, to recall the essence of who they are. When they have finished their assignment they are free to return Home.

Please describe the relationship between the soul and the body.

Without a body the soul is in the realm of unconditional love, and it doesn't have the opportunity to experience anything else. It cannot experience anger, sorrow, or joy of any kind, other than joy of unconditional love. It cannot experience specific kinds of love, such as a child's love; it can only experience the vastness of being in the presence of unconditional love. So it has to have physicality in order to experience any of the physical emotions that you have on planet Earth. These experiences deepen the wisdom of the soul.

Is there any kind of interface between body and soul?

There is a kind of in-between body. This in-between body can be thought of as the prior lessons that the soul has experienced in other bodies. Truthfully, there is no real division; it's more like a physical body growing from childhood into adulthood—the adult isn't different from the child but is just a different aspect of the child. The experience of the child is still there. Such is the way that its experience of past lives remains within the soul itself.

In addition to our soul's memories, does it draw from a greater database of knowledge?

That database is the collective energy where everything is interconnected. So experience of one is the experience of all, but not precisely the same, because you can know the experience of running a four-minute mile, but if you haven't actually done it physically, you don't have the experience of the exertion that it takes. If you observe it occurring, you have the experience that it can be done, and the effort that's needed in order to do it, so in one sense you do have an experience of it, but in another sense, you don't. You could tap into the greater database and draw on that database to discover what you need to know for the physical experience of it.

So what happens when our body dies?
The soul has kept all of the downloaded information. It's like when you buy another computer. If you have all of your files already on one computer, you have to download them into the new computer in order for them to be easily accessible. But you can still retain the original files. So when the soul leaves the body it doesn't make any difference because there's an exact copy. Everything is transferred, with periodic updates. All ideas are energy. Energy is how

21

the information about our life and health is conveyed. In talking in this book about health issues you must never forget that your soul and your body are energy, so all disease and all healing are energy as well. That is of fundamental importance to your understanding what we have to say.

~.~

"Without a body the soul is in the realm of unconditional love, and it doesn't have the opportunity to experience anything else."

The Masters

Section I

On Healing with the Universe

1. Getting Sick

Masters, please describe the fundamental cause of ill health.

Prior to incarnation, the soul itself has determined many different issues that it wishes to experience. Some of these selected experiences may prove so traumatic to the physical body that they can cause energetic blockages within the body which establish diseases of one kind or another.

All diseases begin by our blocking energy, disconnecting from energy, or in some instances even *willing* an adverse change within the body. For instance, some people fixate on cancer, saying that "everybody's got cancer," or "I hope I don't get cancer," or even, "I'm a candidate for this type of cancer." They are going to get cancer because they are calling it into their existence.

Some people actually have, within their physical body, genetic predisposition toward an ailment of one type or another, but this is only a *predisposition*. If a person's ego (which is the conscious, thinking mind) chooses not to follow through with that sensitivity, the body will not develop the condition. But if the ego adopts the attitude that "everybody in the family has it," or (subconsciously) "what will happen will happen" (without the soul being vested in the outcome of that phrase), it will allow the predisposition to come into fruition.

Negativity that some people hold onto disrupts the flow of positive energy into and within the body. If they are constantly fighting the life-force energy, they create blockages that can manifest as any type of physical illness or disease. Conversely, if they make use of the universal life-force energy to help prevent or to break up conditions that have been created by them, they can restore to normal the flow of the energy into and within the body, and rid or even cure themselves of the disruption caused by disease.

Is that the same for little children as for adults?

Mostly young children just let in viruses, energy blockages, and such things because of the vibes they pick up from their parents, such as that "all kids have colds." Also some children may wish to experience what their friends are experiencing. Others wish to be taken care of, and a way to get their parents' full attention is to be sick.

So viruses are real attackers, but are defensible?

Yes. Viruses are like any other living thing in the universe, and like any other energy. You can either invite them to merge with you or tell them to go packing.

How about villagers in Africa facing the deadly Ebola virus in ignorance?

Ignorance is more than just not knowing what's going on. Generally ignorance is accompanied by a layer of fear and a layer of superstition, or the acceptance of the belief systems prevalent in that particular area. An example would be of just blindly believing that "what will happen will happen." This totally obliterates any concept that they can protect themselves from contracting the disease. With the Ebola virus there is superstition, and there is acceptance that "when it comes, everybody gets sick regardless of what you think or do." Such ignorance isn't asking to be sick but sitting back and accepting an opinion about what is "normal."

In respect of that virus you seem to be emphasizing spiritual over physical awareness.

The more people are in contact with their true selves, the more they can dictate, manipulate, and modulate conditions within their human body. This has nothing to do with a person's intellectual powers. Good health is totally up to the soul who possesses the physical body. If an illiterate native believes or knows that he has the power to protect himself because his soul is ultimately powerful, he will not be affected by anything that he does not choose to experience. But if he lets his guard down and listens to those around him, he will be afflicted just as they are.

Some sickness is a result of trauma: an accident, a self-imposed injury, or another person's deliberate act. Do the same principles apply?

What you are referring to are the various ways that a soul may set itself up to deal with desired life lessons. If the lesson is precipitated by an interaction with another human being, then the soul has come into this lifetime with an established contract drawn up with the other soul before their incarnation. The soul was a party to these decisions while in soul form but came down with amnesia concerning the particulars. However, all this pre-planning can still be changed because each soul has freedom of choice.

What about the situation where recovery is remote, when a soldier loses a leg in a battle?

You have to remember that each human life is all about learning lessons and gaining wisdom. If a soul finds itself without an appendage, it is because it has set itself up to learn about overcoming obstacles, self-reliance, self-worth—or even to experience the opposite of each of those traits, such as total helplessness.

If a person has a serious condition with which the human body cannot continue to be viable (dies), it is for one of two reasons. First, the soul may have completed all the lessons it came to earth to experience and wishes to go home to decide his next adventure, or, second, the soul may have made a contract with close human contacts (e.g., parents, sibling, spouse) for them to deal with its departure. Those remaining may need to experience loss, abandonment, betrayal, or feeling guilty that they could have or should have been able to do something to keep the person alive.

What about people with chronic pain which they are desperate to be rid of, but it never goes away?

As hard as it may be for those people to accept, it is their pathway in that lifetime. They are holding onto some lesson that does not allow their body energy to flow smoothly. The lesson may have originated in a previous lifetime. When a lesson is not learned or resolved in one lifetime, souls come back to try again, and again, and again, until they understand what the lesson involves. Unfortunately for the slow learner, the issues get more and more pronounced until the student is aware of them, cannot deny them, and finally gives full attention to the situation or cause. Once the lesson is embraced and dealt with, the soul progresses to the next lesson or, if it is the final lesson of that particular lifetime, returns Home.

2. Getting Well

How effective is self-healing?

Do you mean effective in removing all the restrictions of disease? Or do you mean by easing the soul in its intended purpose for the lesson contained within the disease? Self-healing is very effective in both cases, but they have totally different consequences within the physical body. The first may have the effect of removing every aspect of the disease that is present, while the second may not have any effect on the body itself, but at the soul level it will allow the soul to learn what it wishes to learn.

What can people do to heal themselves of disease?

First, you have to know whether it is for the soul's highest and greatest good that the disease should be removed. If the disease itself is the lesson, *nothing* you do will allow it to be effectively removed. So if a disease is meant to be the lesson or result in the end of that soul's physical life, nothing that you do will reverse the process. When a disease is intended to be a means of learning within a lifetime, you may use the energy of prayer to understand why you chose to have that experience. You have completed that lesson and positive energy can then be used to remove the remaining "debris," which are generally energetic blockages within the body.

Can people use directed thought or prayer to help other people to heal?

Intention is what directs and connects with the energy within the universe.

Directed thought, for a person's highest and greatest good, creates intention. If one directs one's attention to another being, and if the recipient also wishes to learn why he or she has an ailment, then once the reason has been learned, the directed thought definitely has an effect in clearing the residual negative debris. More simply, when the affected person is ready to return to a semblance of normality, their own energy and the energy of their helpers will return the energy within the body to a healthy flow, and the disease within the body will be resolved.

In a situation where someone already has a disease, what is the ideal way of healing?

The ideal way of healing is for the soul to heal itself when it has recognized that it no longer needs the disease. This can be done by a number of different methods that all impact the central energy core of the body, and tap into the universal life-force energies. It can be done by the affected person or by an energy practitioner—someone who has the ability and intention to facilitate the full flow of universal life-force energy. If individuals do not possess the memory of how to use those procedures which stabilize the body, they must rely on a practitioner—because it's all a matter of returning the body to stability. In the case of a virus, bacterium, or invading organism, the body must be returned to a point of balance where the immune system is able to rid the body of any foreign matter.

What of arthritis, for example?

The body is allowing irritants in and an inflammation occurs as a result. This is dealt with by returning the components of the body's immune system to normal. It may be necessary to remove the particular irritant or to desensitize the body to it. Intention and visualization can help one to rearrange and remove irritants.

How about depression?

It depends on the cause of a depression. It can be physical, or coming from a past life, or a spiritual process that the soul is going through as part of a new awareness.

The recognized clinical cause may be from a chemical imbalance, or family difficulties, or the loss of an established behavior pattern. Then the resolution depends upon whatever type of depression it is. In almost every case, the bottom line, so to speak, is the soul's dealing with a spiritual issue that made an imbalance necessary, and that presents what is called a "depressed response to stimuli." Self-healing in these cases is the desire to work through the spiritual lesson.

What about physical things, such as a loss of cartilage?

The body can rebuild itself, and does so constantly. It can be done if the body has the energy to turn on the regeneration process (which most people think shuts off as they age). Just as a lizard can re-grow its tail, a human body can re-grow itself by reactivating the DNA that was turned on at conception to develop the fetus. This provides cells just like our initial healthy cells present at birth. The blueprints of our entire physical system are always stored away and ready to be accessed.

Why did you qualify that remark by saying "if"?
Everything is "if." Everything is up to the soul and what it chooses to do. Frequently the soul within the body is controlled by the ego, the thinking mind. If your ego, from information it has gathered from the world around it, is convinced that because you are a certain age you cannot regenerate something, then you won't be able to regenerate it. It's just like if that same person knows they're going to get cancer because all of their relatives have had cancer, they are going to get cancer.

3. Healing Therapies

Please comment on a list of therapies. Which is the most helpful in getting the healing process going?
It will depend on each individual person and their belief system.

(1) Allopathic (conventional) Medicine?
Allopathic medicine treats the symptoms that are a result of these conditions in the *living shell* of the body caused by the mind's intention or pre-arranged lesson plans.

Medicine alleviates some of the symptoms, but doctors can't really cure anything without the initiative of the soul in reversing those conditions that caused the ailment in the first place. Allopathic medicine can be effective in shifting or turning on and off the bacterial or viral infections which have been allowed into the body either by the soul's invitation or a lack of concern. Repositioning a broken bone so it can be more easily dealt with is in the purview of the doctor. Mostly, however, allopathic medicine masks the symptoms for whatever work the soul needs to do, rather than really effecting a permanent cure. It must be remembered, though, that the circumstances around an illness, such as having to rely on and accept help from others, may themselves be the soul's lesson. And, as we have stated earlier, if a person does not believe that the medicine a doctor is giving them is going to work, it will not.

If a cure follows the use of drugs or radiation, is it because people believe the treatment will cure them?

You are looking at a situation where the person has been presented with a lesson, such as cancer. They realize that the real issue is, say, dealing with their fear of death, and they have resolved that being immortal souls they can never die. Now they have completed the lesson, but they may not be ready to return Home, so they get "cured" to be available to get on to their next lesson. If in dealing with the fear they think they have no escape, and it is either heaven or hell for them, then their physical body collapses under the disease and they cease to exist in a physical form.

(2) Psychiatry, counseling, inspirational techniques (books, films, preachers, motivational speakers)?

All are useful providing that they are geared toward allowing the machinations of the ego to integrate with its spiritual aspects (the heart and soul), and not just mind games where only coping skills are given.

If the practitioners deal with the problem in such a way that the intellect can go inside to feel, analyze, and determine if the thoughts generated are destructive, and if they address those issues and give instructions how to overcome or combat them, then they are excellent. But if the methods are just ways to divert your thinking from one issue to another, they're worthless.

Most inspirational techniques are simply to make people feel good for the moment, and to line the pockets of the speaker! But the inspirational speaker who deals with the power of the soul to manifest, and teaches how to apply the same to physical life, is a self-healing facilitator. Tuning a soul on to its own powers of manifestation allows it to connect with its essence and see the lesson the earthly problems present.

(3) Chinese medicine, acupuncture, Tai Chi, Reiki, and methods of therapeutic touch?

All of them are designed to get people in touch with themselves, and to be aware of what they are doing to themselves and, by doing so, to re-align the processes of their body. It all goes back to the intention of the

37

"healer," who is the person *through whom* energy is being channeled, and also back to the recipient's acceptance and intention. The energy does not come *from* the healing practitioner; he or she is only the facilitator of that energy. This is modulated by the recipients' intention, and at what point they are currently along their path of completing the lesson and understanding the reason for this particular series of events.

With hands-on healing, those who simply channel universal life-force energy do help to align the energies, but they do not impact the cause as directly as the Chinese type of healing does. People who study Tai Chi or Qi Gong can become aware of the energy flow throughout their body in the stillness of the practice. A person who is the subject of manipulation or of energy transfer by another must be open to it, in order for it to work, but develops no more awareness of themselves and what caused their problem.

(4) Emotional Freedom Techniques, Thought Field Therapies?

We have a multi-layered answer. When used as a coping technique or a diversion,

EFT or TFT is like allopathic medicine, just hiding what is going on, but when it is deeply and emotionally felt by a person, so that they get to the root cause of the reason why they are bringing disease within their body, then it is curative. But it is up to the client, who must really get into the causes to effect any change. The therapy is often only as good as the feelings and expansiveness of the person directing it. Do they have the intuitive ability to direct the procedure in such a way that their client really must go inside and make contact with those feelings causing their problems? Or are they only giving the client a coping skill—something to think about—instead of facing and resolving whatever caused the problem in the first place?

(5) Hypnotherapy?

If the client enters hypnosis with an open mind and doesn't fight or try to control what is going on (which can be done even in hypnotic trance), hypnotherapy is excellent, because it is one of the fastest ways to get the person into themselves, in touch with their soul, their higher self, and to get to the root cause of their disease.

What about going into past lives?

Past-life regression allows people to get into things experienced in prior lives, which they have brought forward into the current life because they didn't complete the lesson. Hypnosis allows the intellect to be put on hold so that the feeling heart and soul can come out and report what is holding them hostage. To talk only to the conscious mind will give you a report on what the outside world has convinced the person is true. Talking to the soul or to the higher self (the unconscious mind if you will) taps into the authentic person without outside influence. This is where true awareness begins. Having said this, however, there are qualifiers. The hypnotist must also be a therapist who can feel where the soul is in its journey and must allow the client to direct the procedure and not just implant thoughts or coping skills into that person's subconscious. The entire session needs to be interactive so that the freedom of choice of the client is honored during the process.

Is inter-life regression helpful?

When a person is grappling with the issue of who they are, and why they are currently experiencing the tragedies of this particular life, or when they feel inside that they don't "belong" in this life, allowing them to remember the wisdom of their soul—the time between lives—puts events into perspective. Often they need to seek the wisdom of their individual Council, which helped them to make the decisions that became their life. If they are not ready to have a full immersion in their history (the Akashic records), their higher self will only allow them to connect with what is needed, but however scanty the contact, it answers a lot of questions for the seeker.

How about hypnotic suggestions?

The suggestion type of hypnosis with no input into the particular circumstance of what is going on—unless totally accepted by the person—is of very little value. However, if it is done in a situation where enough information is obtained from the person to pinpoint their problem areas, then it can be effective; but it has to be totally accepted by the person. To say to a hypnotized person that they will cease a particular pattern of behavior will have no lasting effect unless they are predisposed to that action and no longer need the disruption of the particular behavior.

(6) Visualization and creative thoughts?

If visualization is accepted and resonates with people, it lets them direct or participate in their healing, so long as it is done with complete consent and faith in what they are doing. For example, they might be directed to visualize that they have allowed little folk to go into their joints and reconstruct their cartilage. If they don't believe it's possible, it will have no effect. If the helpful little folk are re-seeding and beginning a new growth process, and the people know that this is really possible, then it will have the desired effect.

For skeptics, this may seem a very strange concept, but let us say unequivocally that all souls are in a collective energetic soup. The seasoning that affects any part of the liquid affects all of the soup. If a person can see themselves using the universal energy to heal themselves, they may visualize and accept that the energy can take the form of "little folk," and that in that form it can accomplish the desired task.

(7) Light Language, Vibrational Healing?

These methods go beyond the mind to connect with aspects of the soul that are not totally within the body. The energy involved here makes note of the various imbalances within the body and gives direction back to the lower reaches of the higher self (which are in contact with the body), in order to begin a process of healing.

There must be an acceptance of the lines of communication within the consciousness of the body. If the consciousness does not readily believe, a block to reception will be set up and then nothing will be helpful. Vibrational Healing, Light Language, and crystalline energy all deal with non-visible waveform energy that re-patterns diseases within the body, but negativity or disbelief will stop them cold and prevent their having any restorative action. Using these methods forms a cocoon within which the physical body may rejuvenate if they but bask in the healing energies.

(8) Homeopathy, Flower Essences, Crystals?

The effectiveness of homeopathic remedies is that anything physical that has contact with the body begins the process of changing or stimulating physical elements within the body (rather similar to allopathic medicine), by getting rid of pathogens so that the cause can be corrected. Belief in their effectiveness increases the success of these methods, as it does for allopathic medicine. But if the person does not believe that the medicine given them is going to work, then it will not. A major benefit for the body in the use of these methods is that they do not have toxic effects upon the human system as many chemical allopathic medicines so often do.

Therapies addressing the energy field of the body, rather than its physical aspect, can have a greater effect (such as magnetic, sound, and vibrational modalities), because these affect not only the physical but also the etheric field containing the history that is carried on from lifetime to lifetime which frequently determines a predisposition for sensitivity to disease or imbalance. It can also bring into consciousness the cause of the disruption.

4. Weight Loss Issues

Is it correct that we all have a natural weight?

What you are referring to is a genetic predisposition, if the body is left to its own devices. This predisposition has to do with your thoughts, your eating habits, your metabolism, your hidden motivations, and the way the food is utilized. In order to really change the composition of your body you have to take positive action by rewriting existing hidden programs (physical genetics) within the body. Most people don't go that far. They will experiment with a new diet, exercise program, or even use an appetite suppressant. Then they relax and their old default genetic predisposition programming takes over again and they are right back where they started. Then, to safeguard their position, the hidden programs generally add additional weight as a protection against depletion in the future.

Is that like having a computer program inside you, where you can actually re-write the default?

Yes, precisely. Basically a person does this by pattern modification. The genetics of the body create a pattern for the physical activity within the body, for its metabolism, taste, et cetera. "Taste" is the insatiable predisposition for sugars, starches, and the like. If people ever cease to have intentional modification of their default programming, the program becomes dominant again. If they consciously take the effort to first rewrite the taste program and then increase their activity level, they are able to change the default, which results in weight loss.

Taste and the activity level are central?

They are the two keys. Taste, of course, goes into all of the non-nutritional as well as

46

the nutritional food stuff, and exercise burns off excess fat while building lean muscle mass, so that food is used more efficiently. People can rewrite their body's defaults with hypnosis, but they must have the intention to do so.

Can they use meditation?

They can have the thought given to them in hypnosis. They can give it to themselves in meditation, but with either means of introduction, they still have to become self-disciplined and follow through. The concept of behavior modification can't be something that is just put there in the back of the mind and not integrated. It must have a personalized motivational trigger to fire it, because the conscious mind is so strong that it really must be totally reprogrammed. This generally presents itself as a reward, such as improved health or a fantastic body which can be fit into "normal" size clothing.

So a little brainwashing is necessary?

[Laughing] Yes, in a manner of speaking.

If I understand correctly, in order to get Mr. and Mrs. Tubby to slim down they must have three things: rigorous discipline, supportive hypnosis, and group work where they get excited about change.

The intention to change and implement the means necessary to achieve weight loss is the discipline. Hypnosis or meditation is the primer. Group work is very important because that motivates the continuation of the other two. Weight loss is not easy but it can be done.

What is a realistic goal?

Caution must be taken not to lose weight as far as possible because people can go beyond a healthy percentage of fat for the sake of the body, saying, "I'm going to get rid of this fat so I'll never put it back on!" Then they go overboard and start losing muscles and doing other harm. The right way is to do it very gradually, with behavior modification, so that they find what is comfortable for their skeletal framework— not what they see through their eyes but what they physically feel is the best for them. For some people it may be a slim body, for others a compact physique that might be considered to be overweight by some but which, for both their bone and their muscular structure, is perfectly normal. Each person seeking weight loss must find their ideal proportion.

What about the search in hypnotic regression for trigger points—the initial sensitizing events of severe stress resulting in unconscious gorging?

That's very important. These events give a predisposition to the body to add unneeded weight. There are also the spiritual and psychological reasons which have caused the individual to modify and re-enforce the genetic predisposition to be overweight. What you do, after the fact, is to attempt both to modify the genetic predispositions and to clear out all the unconscious issues that are keeping them implanted. These may include such events as an early present-life where they were starving, so now they are storing up as much extra body fat as they possibly can; or a past life where people who weren't fat were not considered to be prosperous or healthy.

49

Many events, such as these, have strong spiritual and psychological ties which are hard to break, as well as tending to activate a physical predisposition or a safety statement "I need more weight." So there can be a dual curative purpose when you go back to an initial sensitizing event.

The "I am starving" routine is where they started gorging and packing on fat, and it can be analyzed for the effect it now has, and an evaluation can be made to rewrite the result in terms of an erroneously perceived danger. In essence, let them come to the realization that this predisposition is an abnormal one for them given the current situation. Let their subconscious choose, while in hypnosis (outside the reach of their conscious mind), to have a more efficient body.

How do we modify a genetic predisposition—by talking it away somehow?

You have to rewrite it. It is like when you have a tendency to do something, you can make the choice not to do it. As we have said before about a person with a genetic predisposition for cancer, such as all the members of their family being afflicted: if all their talk is, "I'm going to get cancer," they will, but if they say instead "I'm going to take control of my energy to make sure it doesn't get blocked, so I don't get cancer," that is changing the genetic predisposition.

The same with weight and body mass, if the individual's predisposition is for a huge body mass, it is going to come about unless there are actions taken: "I don't have to have that body mass." "I choose to activate that part of my metabolism which will regulate the body mass." "I don't have to have this sluggish metabolism." "I don't have to have this total blockage, packing on fat cells like this." "I can have a normal proportion because I choose to balance my body."

Will this actually reverse the fat cells that are always hungry for more?

Yes, it will gradually change the way that everything within the body interprets the nourishment that is put into the body, how it is utilized, and in what form it is stored. When the cells find they can function with

less than they used to ingest, they will see no
need to keep gorging.

~.~

"The intention to change and
implement the means necessary
to achieve weight loss is the
discipline. Hypnosis or meditation
is the primer. Group work is very
important because that motivates
the continuation of the other two.
Weight Loss is not easy but it can
be done."

The Masters

The Soul's Creative Power

Masters, in what other ways may an individual incarnated soul use its creative powers?

There are two distinct aspects of the soul's creative powers. One is the creative power of intention; the other is the creative power of the physical application of the intention. For example, a person must have the intention to obtain a degree in order to become a doctor or a lawyer. That is the intention—the energy she puts into the discipline of doing whatever it takes to fulfill her desire. This includes all the aspects of certainty within herself that she can carry the desired action to completion. This creates a waveform in which she already sees herself at the destination. Then she must also have the physical manifestation, such as her personal involvement in applying to be accepted by the professional school. Having completed the prerequisites, then she has to come up with the money in order to be able to afford the school. That is how she puts her intention into physical manifestation. She cannot just sit back and expect that the universe will arrange all the human physical factors, simply because she has put the intention out there.

If people only have the intention on a spiritual level to go forward with something but don't take the physical steps needed to set it up, they will not complete it. So *manifestation* does not mean a person only has to dream or think and it is so.

Can individual souls really change the vibrational frequency at which they live?

Without a doubt. The way to accomplish the task is by cleaning their spiritual house. By Spiritual House we refer to the state of consciousness of the soul level that they are able to maintain, divorcing themselves from the day-to-day ego level of human life. It is the act of ridding themselves of their fears, doubts, and negativity.

An example would be where two people have recently divorced. If they remain in bitterness, in loss of expectation, and all the negative feelings which caused them to realize they had to divorce in the first place, they are in a very low vibrational state and will be angry, agitated, and tired all the time. If they choose to detach themselves from those feelings, because they are not needed and serve no purpose, realizing that it was just something that happened so they could learn a lesson, then they can cut loose and move on.

They will begin to restore vitality as they detach from each energy (you'd call it a memory, but it is an energy that is there). If they get rid of the photos that remind them, if they no longer fixate on their former spouse, then, instead, they will look forward to a life for themselves and with themselves, connecting with the energy inside of them.

This is important, because having rid themselves of outside stimulation from their former spouse, they need to find inside stimulation. They need to find love somewhere or they will go back to the same type of situation from which they just removed themselves.

All human beings can connect with the unconditional love that is in their soul while still in physical form. Each little increment of a physical being connecting with a tiny spark of that unconditional love changes their vibration. When they are able to connect totally with that energy, they are completely removed from negativity and are in unconditional love almost to the extent of being in the pure spiritual form. The end result is an increase in vibrational frequency.

~.~

"If people only have the intention on a spiritual level to go forward with something but don't take the physical steps needed to set it up, they will not complete it."

The Masters

Comment

While people say "a good mental attitude helps us to heal," most of us also believe that a specific healing method helps to cure us of disease. The Masters go a lot further. They say that the only effective way of healing a person's ailments is when their soul's specific intention to heal works in and through their physical body. This intention to heal may well be helped by the activity of a healing practitioner, and supported by the energy and prayers sent to a sick person by other people, but *only* the soul's positive attitude, transmitted through their authentic intent and practical creativity, is effective. Viruses may be destroyed and bones may be reset, but only the soul will actually provide the energy for healing the body.

They also spoke of dealing with the initial cause or reason why the soul chose to have the experience. We need to know whether an affliction is a lesson we can complete by overcoming it and moving on, or if we must grapple with it for the duration of our physical life.

We included paragraphs from the Masters on "The Soul's Creative Powers" in order to put this very specific teaching into context. Each of us possesses an eternal soul who has chosen to enter into our body shell to face, and often to endure, a variety of experiences from which valuable lessons may be learned. Before it comes down to Earth, the soul makes these choices to gain wisdom and develop maturity. Our spirit is a loving being, always in contact with the unconditional love of the universe flowing from the Source. But it has the difficult task of working through the physical body and coping with the strong, controlling ego of the conscious mind that gets us into trouble and often censures our better judgments. So it is only when we allow ourselves to recognize and connect with our eternal soul that we can truly change the vibrations in our body from negative to positive, and allow in the enabling, healing energy that we need to live healthy, happy lives.

Sickness generally comes to us from our mind's ignorant, or even willful decisions. We can grasp this idea when we see a young person injured while playing a dangerous sport. It is much harder to understand such a concept when holding a colicky baby!

The Masters recognize that many health issues are pre-arranged experiences to test us. Some we may be able to overcome, but some frailties remain with us until the day we die. Then there are other illnesses which come in solely because we permit them, or even because we invite them. These we can overcome by our soul's intention, acted upon in a way that is consistent with a true intention. Thus our soul, which is always filled with the healing energy of the Creator's universal love, can direct healing into our body and we will be cured.

Despite their words, many people may feel uncertain what to do next. To help us to overcome this difficulty the Masters give advice. Healing practitioners can aid our return to health if we are willing to trust what they do. But we should look beyond our trust in the healer of our choice. What we must do is to exercise our intention to heal our body, having "the intention on a spiritual level to go forward," and so take the physical steps needed to do so. But we remember that we can do this on our own.

We can attract good health to ourselves:
1. By having the goal of good health in our mind.
2. By holding a firm intention and taking positive steps to reach that goal.
3. By censoring and contradicting every single negative thought and action which is contrary to that goal.
4. By expressing gratitude for every positive sign of progress that comes to us.
5. By accepting renewed good health when it comes back into our life.

So, with or without the help of a healer, if the soul signals that we can rid ourselves of our sickness because it does not represent a long-term experience we chose in advance (and we will know if that is the case), then we may be healed of all those diseases which are capable of being reversed. We have the Masters' word for that.

Section II

On Meditation

Masters, how effective is meditation in enhancing the soul's spiritual awareness?

On planet Earth, the word Meditation is used in a number of ways. There is no set definition of what it is. That said, if you are engaged in a meditation which is aimed at making you feel better, or reducing stress, or putting you into a peaceful mood, it does nothing for you other than deal with your physical issues. You will learn to breathe properly and to control some of your bodily functions, such as blood pressure and heart rate, but as a spiritual discipline it will be ineffective.

From a spiritual viewpoint, meditation is truly a form of communication that can exist between your soul and the rest of the souls in the universe. If you use meditation to prepare yourself for this communication by bringing out aspects of your humanity and unlearned prior lessons from past lives, and if you go inside and dig around for blockages which you have put in your way, and remove them so they are not a part of your consciousness and are not hanging on to what the energy of your soul is trying to accomplish, then you reach a state of bliss.

You must come to a state of understanding that the soul in its purest form cleanses the residuals of human nature, clarifies your spiritual purpose or pathway, and authenticates the spirit within the human body which exists as unconditional love. When you have reached this awareness you may dialogue with the other souls within that pure, clear, unaffected space. This is the enlightened purpose of meditation.

Physically, once that state is reached, your meditation brings you from the outside world into a place where soul communicates to soul. Then you can tap into the wisdom of the universe and within that state bring forth that wisdom to complete whatever purpose you have for being on the planet.

On Prayer

Masters, I need guidance about a friend asking me to pray for someone injured in a car crash.

Most people think that our futures are predetermined and that we are but puppets of some force outside of us, instead of knowing that each individual soul has the ability to create its own reality. When people ask for prayers, it is because they are fearful as they feel forsaken by whatever energy is outside of them (such as their god), and because they do not want to be responsible for themselves. If they believe that someone "out there" calls the shots, then they do not have to be responsible for themselves. All blame can be assigned elsewhere.

The prayers requested were for someone else.

That does not matter because a person who requests prayer relates to the situation, putting herself into the same position and wondering if she would be able to be saved.

63

There is that edge of despair, so "let's stay on the good side of that force outside of us" and, in that same vein, we can help our friend by being an intermediary between that force, the self, and the person.

Requesting another to pray is like saying that two are better than one, three are better than two—that volume makes a difference.

Are you saying that prayer does not make any difference?

It depends on your definition of prayer. To the majority of people, praying is making a request for intervention for help, to be bailed out of what is perceived as a helpless, hopeless situation.

Is it not effective?

In that respect it is not effective. Instead, if what is sent to the universe is *gratitude* for allowing us, and any person for whom our prayers have been requested, to experience what we need to experience, it reinforces that person's intention by adding energy to it and aids in completing that person's particular lesson.

Was their soul's intention to have the car crash?

It was to experience the outcome of that incident and to learn from it. The soul set itself up to experience a human lesson, and as it came to pass, the way to accomplish that lesson was to be involved in a car crash or something similar.

Does that mean that the soul knew in advance what the outcome would be?

The soul didn't know the exact outcome; it only knew that it would be presented with a physical situation which would allow it to experience the lesson. An example could be that as a result of the car crash a woman was crippled. She would experience helplessness and the need to ask other people for aid. If she also experienced some type of mental affliction as a result of the accident, she would have to overcome that impairment, which did not exist before. The precise incident is not always known in advance, only whether it is going to be helplessness, hopelessness, or being able to rebuild after having been torn apart. So the basic lesson plan is established, not the specific lesson.

Is there any means (such as sending positive energy or meditating) by which an outsider can affect the outcome of the incident?

Yes. If the person who is undergoing the lesson has, say, a broken leg and will have to go through life without being able to maneuver easily, any healing energy sent to him (if he is willing to receive it) will let him understand that both his attitude and reception of such energy can hasten his return to health. It also allows people in such a situation to learn about their own creative powers, and the increase of the energy supplied by others illuminates their situation, allowing them to see it more readily.

Many people send energy to the patient by praying: "I pray that their suffering will be alleviated." This translates energetically as, "Let them understand this lesson they have chosen so that they do not have to continue experiencing it but can heal and move on."

If it is possible to affect an outcome, is it necessarily for the best to try to do so? Will the universe simply disallow it if it doesn't serve the highest good?

The universe doesn't "disallow" anything. What happens is that the recipient of the energy, the victim or patient, may choose not to receive it. This may be either because in his present state he does not believe that help can be had from any outside source other than allopathic medicine, antibiotics, bone grafts, or things of that nature, or because he feels that he deserves to be in his present situation for some perceived wrong that he may have done. Most of the time when energy of this kind does not work, it is because the recipient refuses to allow the energy to come in and aid him, or he is not ready for his highest and greatest good to move on at that time.

Is such refusal at a soul level?

Sometimes this refusal for help is even at a conscious level. If the healer is, say, a chiropractor or an acupuncturist who is not accepted by the person, or a reiki master and the recipient doesn't believe in all "that energy nonsense," then proffered energy definitely will not work. If then the universe is asked to intervene it will not do so because that would be interfering with the lessons to be learned and the person's free will to reject any offered assistance.

Some people say they can feel or sense the prayers of others and find comfort or healing in them. Is this wishful thinking or (rather than traditional prayer) are they actually sensing the elevated vibrations of good and loving thoughts directed their way?

In an open-minded soul the latter is true. They are cognizant of the fact that energy is being supplied to them, particularly if they are in a depleted condition because they allowed their energy to slip away, or they have given it up by worrying about causes that have nothing to do with the problems they are going through. They can be replenished by the energy of others, which they may perceive as the prayers of well-wishers.

Where the intention coming from the person who is assisting their recovery is one of providing energy for the highest good of the soul—if the soul is open to it—then the recipient will perceive a feel-good situation, and, if they are open enough to it, they may even feel the mending of a broken bone. A person undergoing acupuncture can sense not only energy being transmitted along the meridians from needle to needle, but also the acupuncturist's intention, adding an extra zing to those needles, because he is giving of his own energy to facilitate the overall healing.

Positive vibrations have been shown to affect the condition of plants and animals, as well as humans. Can we assume that directing loving attentions toward someone works to their advantage, or at least does no harm?

[Laughter] Absolutely! Universal healing energy comes with a guarantee that it will only apply itself for the highest and greatest good. Universal energy is unconditional love that cannot and never does harm a living thing.

What is the best way to send loving positive energy?

Connect yourself to the feel of the energy of the universe; you will sense that you are connected to all that exists, physical and non-physical. Then direct that energy to the person you wish to assist, intending that, for the highest and greatest good (as they, not the universe, determine), they may be aided in their lesson. This lets individuals decide if they have completed that particular lesson and may move on or if they have to continue in like manner.

When you use the term "universe," what exactly do you mean?

We use the term "universe" to portray everything that is not the individual energy of the particular soul you are assisting—so it is the totality of all other energy outside of that one particular soul. Many call this the God-Force or Source, which is part and parcel of all souls. Everything is energy and energy is everything.

Please outline the steps by which human beings may connect "to the feel of the energy of the universe."

First, and most importantly, the easiest way to do that is for people to have a feel for their self—to know themselves. In order for this to happen, they must be without fear, they must be without doubt, they must have a sense and a knowing that they are part of the universe of all that is. For those who have not previously experienced this to synchronize with the universe, they must start by acknowledging that all souls come from one Source, and therefore we are all one and the same. Acknowledging that fact, it becomes easy for each to say, "I am going to connect to the rest of myself." The rest of oneself is, of course, the universe.

How do they then direct that energy to a person they wish to assist?

Simply, it is effected by the intention they have for the direction of the energy. If, for example, a person wants to heal an animal but their intention is for everything in the universe to be balanced, then the energy they are connecting to and directing will be dissipated throughout the universe. Instead, if their concentration is for energy needed to bring that specific animal into balance, and it is directed to the animal, it will be as if they are taking an intensification cone and funneling the energy to that one animal. It is the same with a person, it is the same with a plant, it is even the same with an inanimate object, with everything needing a little help to come into balance.

~.~

"Universal healing energy comes with a <u>guarantee</u> that it will only apply itself for the highest and greatest good. Universal energy is unconditional love that cannot and never does harm a living thing."

The Masters

Prayer in the Christian Bible *(Revised Standard Version)*

The Masters use the phrase: "The Third Dimension." Their view is of the universe being composed of strata, ascending levels or bands of energetic vibration, similar to low frequency sound waves compared with higher frequency light waves. All these levels coexist but, as in a radio receiver, you can tune to only one at a time for truly clear reception. Third Dimension describes the lower vibrational level of planet Earth and all her natural life, including human beings. This level is ruled primarily by the ego, the thinking, plotting mind, and by the belief systems that must be accepted for membership in society. The fourth and higher dimensions refer to the higher vibrations of the spirit world where the heart and feelings rule from the experiences of the soul. Each soul creates its own reality based upon the collective wisdom. Here there is no duality so there is no fear or doubt, only a sense of "knowing."

The Masters survey our society from the perspective of their spiritual Home in the positive realm of unconditional love. They look at a world which is polarized not just physically as a globe, but more importantly between the positive and the negative, good and evil, rich and poor, and so on. Yet, at the same time, each human being contains within its shell an entirely positive and loving immortal soul who belongs to the God-Force, composed of all souls in the universe. Souls come to Earth in order to experience a variety of chosen lessons during their time in physical form. Learning about the nature of prayer is one of the practical applications of such lessons.

The Masters on the Bible

The Masters asked to comment on 12 biblical references to prayer in order to help some readers. We made the selection.

The Lord's Prayer

Jesus says in Matthew 6: 9-13:
"Pray then like this:
Our father who art in heaven,
Hallowed be thy name .
Thy kingdom come, Thy will be done,
On earth as it is in heaven.
Give us this day our daily bread;
And forgive us our debts
as we also have forgiven our debtors;
And lead us not into temptation,
But deliver us from evil."

The Lord's Prayer came at a time when people really needed to feel they belonged to something. They needed also to believe that they were protected, and had someone responsible for those things over which they had no control. The Prayer let them know there was something (which was a part of them) outside of themselves. In general, people think kindly of their parents. Parents are our protectors, guides, and directors with whom we feel secure and safe. The words *Our father who art in heaven* indicate that part of us truly is also outside of us, outside of the physical "shell" with which we identify ourselves. When people feel their true essence, they can feel that the energy outside themselves is inside them as well—it is within their soul.

The majority of the prayer defines how a soul is to comport itself during the period of time when it is within a physical being. The prayer is less instructive today than in an age when communication was not as prevalent. It told people who were illiterate to be part of the whole. The translation here, though accepted by most sects, is not of the words which were originally given…

Not even the Greek version we have?

Not even the Greek. Bled into it were the ideologies of the male-dominated society of the time, where it was important for men to be in charge; therefore, the address it made was to the "Father."

The prayer had roots in Jewish prayers, didn't it?

It had many sources, Jewish and even older. The concept of our being connected to something outside of us permeates the whole prayer. Its entire energy speaks of the soul being universal and of it being broken off from and identified with the Source. This prayer is a reminder—providing the energy of the prayer is felt—that we are everything that exists, and that we should honor not only that energy within us, but that energy within all of those around us, and know that we belong to a place of unconditional love, wherein all are equal, which totally accepts and adheres to loving and providing all that is.

In modern terminology you would refer to this prayer as an affirmation. It asks that all our energy, that contained inside of our selves in combination with that which remains outside in the universe (which we acknowledge and honor as the divine aspect of ourselves), combine to take care of our earthly physical needs while we continue on in these bodies. Let us learn from the lessons that we have undertaken so that we do not have to repeat those that caused discomfort, even as we give gratitude for those that have helped us on this journey.

The Gloria

Praise, based on Revelation 4: 8-9 & 11:
"Glory be to the Father and to the Son and to the
Holy Spirit. As it was in the beginning, is now,
and ever shall be, world without end."

This prayer is a mantra, a celebration, a thankfulness for the individual identity of each one of us, and that we also are, in essence, "everything." It is in the vernacular that people used to give praise, but it says "glory to us, glory to who we are, because we are all of this."

The indirect reference to the Trinity is to the power of our physical being connecting with our spiritual being, which connects with all that is. That is the power of the Trinity, the most forceful energy anywhere, and it is eternal, never ending. It represents the energy of that which is broken off from the Source (*Father*) into the human (*Son*), with its connection to the parts of us that are still in the spiritual realm (*Holy Spirit*), and the force it then creates with its new wisdom as it reunites back with Source.

The Hail Mary

A petition broadly based on Luke 1: 28 and 42:
Hail Mary, full of grace,
The Lord is with thee.
Blessed art thou amongst women,
And blessed is the fruit of thy womb, Jesus.
Holy Mary, Mother of God,
Pray for us sinners, now
And at the hour of our death.

There's a lot going on in this mantra (we say mantra, not prayer, because it re-affirms who we are at the spiritual level).

Hail Mary honors the feeling side of the physical, the feminine side, acknowledging that all souls contain both male and female energy. It is within the female role that we truly feel and appreciate life, and we birth the male experience. The male comes forth, and the true physical experience, which is within the ego, can begin. There's also an admonition in this prayer not to enter into or go beyond sinful ways in ignorance of who you are, but always to come back to the union between the energies of the soul.

Jesus' last words from the cross

From Luke 23: 34
"Father, forgive them,
For they do not know what they do."

This is an acknowledgement that, within the physical (due to contracts we have set up to allow us to experience things), deeds are done in the third dimension which are classified as "right" and "wrong." In Earth's dimension people go into an arena of blame. To assuage the energy of our thoughts that someone has done us wrong, the only thing which can bring us back into balance, harmony, and unconditional love is forgiveness. The person who has gone through the experience of suffering wrong in the third dimension is the only one who can release that energy by forgiving the transgressor.

This is also a skewed rewrite of thoughts that were said at that time. Jesus was quoted as having called upon the Father to forgive, presumably so that the souls of his tormentors would not be condemned to Hell. The request that was directed to the

"Father" refers to that judgmental Supreme Power outside of self that made all the decisions and meted out all the punishments. This also alludes to the fact that although you made the contracts to do certain things before you incarnated, when you actually entered into the body you had total amnesia.

From Luke 23: 46
"Father, into your hands I commend my spirit!"

This prayer of gratitude is for what others allow us to experience. It is a prayer of recognition that we all come from the same Source and return to the same Source. Or, in today's vernacular, "I'm coming Home!"

Job's cry of anguish

Job 1: 20
"Naked I came from my mother's womb, and naked shall I return. The Lord gave and the Lord has taken away; blessed be the name of the Lord."

How drama sells in the third dimension! Human feelings have to contain the sense of what is right or wrong. In this verse, the lament of Job's soul is, in effect, "I came down here to the physical without any knowledge of who I was. If I stay without any knowledge of who I am, I will not have grown as a soul, until I return and then I can look back and see what was accomplished."

So this is a plea to go inside, connect with your essence, connect with the God-Force which (without your knowledge) you feel only exists outside you, and then recognize that which lies within you to obtain true experience and develop true wisdom.

Examples of how to pray

Mark 11: 24-25 are words of instruction by Jesus: "Therefore I tell you, whatever you ask in prayer, believe that you receive it, and you will."

This is an outline of how the human, physical experience exists on Earth, showing that we all come down with our God-Force energy, with the ability to use the power of manifestation. Then, with our intention, we can create the reality or the circumstances that we need to experience, and we begin the process of learning the experiences we need in order to grow.

Recently other people have spoken about this principle which you call "The Law of Attraction." It translates into the fact that what you intend or fixate on is created. This works both for the things that you want and the things you fear. If you spend time intending to advance at work you will create an energy that will "return" to you in this case as a promotion. If you spend all your time worrying about getting fired, your actions will show that you have little concern for your job, so it is terminated.

Matthew 26:39 are words from Jesus' prayer in the garden of Gethsemane:
"My Father, if it be possible, let this cup pass from me; nevertheless not as I will, but as thou wilt."

These words are an acknowledgment that we should always be aware of the fact that we have freedom of choice. However, we remind ourselves that we have begun upon a path and have created experiences for our journey down that path before ever we began this lifetime. This still allows our physical self to ask why we wanted such an experience in the first place. We ask our God-self, "Why did I do this? Isn't there some other way I can do it?" And of course, because we have freedom of choice the answer is "Yes." But if we opted out of the experience this time around, in order to have the experience we chose, we would then need to come back and do it over again in another form. Jesus also acknowledged that while his physical self (ego/mind) did not like the idea of his future, his spiritual self (heart/soul) had chosen the experience.

1 John 3: 21-22
"Beloved, if our hearts do not condemn us, we have confidence before God; and we receive from him whatever we ask, because we keep his commandments and do what pleases him."

A total misconception, and one where it was something construed to give control to the religious leaders. Translation: "I am a good and obedient person who does not want to make decisions, so please take all of my power and responsibility away from me, and in exchange take care of my needs."

We have within us the divine power to manifest and to create. If we cut ourselves off from our knowledge, our feelings, and the wisdom of our power, if we do not accept responsibility for the ability we have, we will seek it outside ourselves, and then we cannot and will not learn.

We must return to balance, to an understanding, knowledge, and wisdom of the divinity within us, of who we are. When we have faith and trust in ourselves, then all can be completed.

1 Peter 3:12
"For the eyes of the Lord are upon the righteous and his ears are open to their prayer. But the face of the Lord is against those who do evil."

This raises a totally different issue which makes perfect sense if you take it within the realm of the third dimension, the duality of the physical world. If you take it into the spiritual realm it makes no sense at all, as there is nothing but unconditional love with no judgment present here. This verse seeks to help assuage the doubts and justify people in the third dimension in taking care of themselves and their wants. As long as they comply with the belief systems of their society, everything they do will be righteous. Again, this presents a control issue. It ceases to make any sense as we raise up our physical self to the soul level.

Isn't there another aspect when souls deliberately choose to do what the world calls "Evil" as a lesson?
You are right, and they would be totally condemned by this verse, and truly they are condemned within the third dimension, the area of judgment, because the duality on the

planet is both positive and negative. Within the realm of the higher dimensions they are exalted for their choice that allows extremes to be felt. The positive cannot exist on Earth without the negative, and vice versa. In the spirit realm, there is no duality. Those who have chosen to experience negativity allow us spirits to feel the greatness of the unconditional love in which we exist, but in fact, without their feeling the depth of depravity (the negativity of the third dimension), we would not know the extent of such magnificence.

1 Thessalonians 5: 16-18
"Rejoice always, pray constantly, give thanks in all circumstances; for this is the will of God in Christ Jesus for you."

This is a mantra of recognition of who you are. Affirm who you are, rejoice in who you are, and be grateful when you recognize and when you connect with who you are. If you do this you will bring the energy that others think is outside of you, into you, and so you will live that life upon the earth. This is the path of the soul.

James 1:5-8
"If any of you lacks wisdom, let him ask God, who gives to all men generously and without reproaching, and it will be given him. But let him ask in faith, with no doubting, for he who doubts is like a wave of the sea that is driven and tossed by the wind. For that person must not suppose that a double-minded man, unstable in all his ways, will receive anything from the Lord."

This is about the law of attraction. This is about the battle between the soul (the heart energy, the healing energy), and the ego (the earthbound energy). This is trusting and discovering who you are. This is allowing yourself to tap into the wisdom that you have gained in past experiences, past lives, past connections with those in the spirit world, bringing your God-self into your physical being, and letting it permeate your very existence. On a physical level this enables you to accept who you are, and to have faith that the knowledge you gained in the past gives you wisdom you can apply in this lifetime. This can happen only if you don't let those around you, who created your ego by telling you what they want you to think and believe, take control. If you follow the ego which constantly battles for earthly prominence, it will overshadow the power, the knowledge, the acceptance, and the connection of who you truly are. During an incarnation your soul's intention will always be to become your true authentic self, your soul expression in human form. Accept it, have faith in it, and let it direct you to further wisdom that can be gained in the physical experience.

~.~

"When a people feel their true essence, they can feel that the energy outside themselves is inside them as well—it is within their soul."   *The Masters*

Comment

The Masters see traditional prayer, the type people learn at Sunday School, as being ineffective. The reason for this will be quite new for most of us. It is that there are no true accidents in our lives, because all souls follow a path filled with experiences that represent the lessons we have agreed to in advance of coming down to planet Earth. Therefore we should understand why the universe is not going to take away any of our lessons from us merely because we don't like an experience at the last moment and plead for help. That would void our prior agreement, which we carefully thought out and freely made before we came down to planet Earth, and interfere with our soul's essential freedom of choice.

So can anything be done to help us? Yes. We can use the energetic power that lies within each one of us to encourage our growth in understanding and wisdom, and to aid our self-healing. We can be truly open to the methods, energy, and unspoken prayers of skilled healing practitioners. We can be receptive to the healing energy that others may choose to send us. We can learn to understand our own energetic make up, and know when it is out of balance so that we may return it to stability before disease takes over.

When there are other people who want to come to our aid, through their intention they can redirect the positive energy of the universe, which is always freely available for them to use as channels of loving energy, to aid our further healing. Their expression of gratitude for our life lessons is the gift they may beam to us, from near or far, to enrich and strengthen the energy of our soul.

Knowing the Masters' overall point of view will help our better understanding of their unique Bible-study commentary. They told us that their intention was to give people a feeling that the ideas they cling to cannot always be interpreted in the light of (what they call) "modern" thinking. They also commented more personally, "If these verses and thoughts are taken into the soul and truly felt, and if you tap into the wisdom that is within your higher self, you will know how this will help you better understand the human experience you are having."

For believing Christians, Muslims, and Jews, the idea of God as someone who is *wholly other* than themselves is central to their religious thinking. God is seen as the one *from whom* they receive and *to whom* they turn. To some people the very thought of God being *within* the human soul itself smacks of blasphemy. For such, the very idea that the human soul is a small part of the almighty Creator is anathema. Yet, however we judge the Masters' biblical commentary, it is based on the following concepts:

- "God," whom they call *Creator* or *Source*, is the unconditional love whose energy fills the whole of the universe.

- The Creator "broke off" from itself a myriad of energetic *souls* who remain as particles of universal unconditional love, yet they are afforded individuality and free will in order to enhance the wisdom of the whole God-Force in which they exist.

- Individual souls have the opportunity to deepen their understanding of the nature of unconditional love by incarnating on planet Earth, which is a dimension of total energetic polarization between the positive and negative.

- When each soul incarnates it has amnesia as to who it was, and why it has become what it now is. This is so that it may rediscover, from lessons it undertakes in human physicality, its true identity as a fragment of the divine.

- Our return Home to the spiritual realm will involve our making a self-review of the life-lessons we experienced while on Earth. This review will not involve our being judged by other spirits for our success or failure, however, because such judgment is wholly absent in the unconditional love of the place where we all belong.

So, here the Masters of the Spirit World explain their approach, which we can see is significantly different from that commonly advanced by existing religions, but they are truly understanding of our needs and are completely without blasphemy. We may choose to reject their reasoning—after all we have free will, as they often say. In these studies we believe that open-minded people will find a true coherence and the radiance of unconditional love and service of our needs.

If this book is your first venture into understanding the ways of the soul, please be patient. Understanding what the Masters have to say may not come overnight.

The world is going through a time of real crisis in our generation, and it is good for each one of us to find out who we are at the deepest level of our existence.

In these books we are creating for the Masters, and on the website where they will address us weekly, they hope to give further encouragement and help to you for your journey through life.

The Authors

The Reverend Peter Watson Jenkins, MA (Cantab.), LLB, CH, works as a clinical and metaphysical master hypnotist, specializing in past-life regression and spirit release. In the 1960s he studied theology at Cambridge University (UK), and was a parish minister for 21 years. He lectures on reincarnation, and has written the following books:

> *Escape to Danger* (2001) (as *Watson Jenkins*)
> *Training for the Marathon of Life* (2005)
> *Talking with Leaders of the Past* (2007)
> *Christy's Journey Through 12 Past Lives* (2008)

Toni Ann Winninger, JD, CH, is a Reiki master and is well established as a psychic channeler. She also works as a metaphysical hypnotist, practices spirit release, and teaches metaphysical subjects, including Light Language. Before the Masters called her to become a channeler, she worked as a prosecutor for the Cook County State's Attorneys' Office, in Chicago, Illinois, USA.

Toni (President) and Peter (CEO) are officers of Celestial Voices, Inc. publishers of this book.

Visit the Masters' Website

www.MastersOfTheSpiritWorld.com

- Read the Masters' weekly message.
- Sign up for the Newsletter
- Give the Masters your feedback
- Tell everybody.

Celestial Voices, Inc.

This book was published by Celestial Voices Inc., a Chicago-based company. We hope that what you just read proves to be of lasting value for you. We invite readers to consider sharing the Masters' wisdom by purchasing more copies of this book. This can be done by logging on to our website:

www.CelestialVoicesInc.com

On this site you will find details of the other publications Peter Watson Jenkins has written with Toni Ann Winninger, and news of the work they are doing to promote the wisdom and loving celestial voices of the Masters of the Spirit World.